THE APHASIA SERIES

VOLUME ONE

SFA, RET, AND RAP

MARIA L. MUÑOZ, PH.D., CCC-SLP

RECIPE SLP

The Aphasia Series, Volume One, SFA, RET, and RAP

Copyright © 2014 by Maria L. Muñoz

This book is published by
Recipe SLP
Fort Worth, TX
http://www.recipeslp.com

Cover design by Seth Hepler
Formatting by RikHall.com

Print version - ISBN:978-1-941352-04-5
Kindle version - ISBN:978-1-941352-03-8

Contents

SEMANTIC FEATURE ANALYSIS

(SFA)

Semantic Feature Analysis (SFA)

Purpose:

SFA improves the lexical retrieval of nouns by strengthening and/or restoring activation within the semantic system. An organizational chart is used to elicit semantic features in order to stimulate the activation required to produce a target word.

Researchers have reported outcomes for a number of variations of SFA. This guide focuses on SFA procedures that encourage patients to *generate* the features of nouns. Separate Recipe SLP guides will address SFA procedures that emphasize the recognition of semantic features or target other grammatical classes.

Intended Population:

SFA is designed for individuals with anomia and may benefit patients with no more than a moderate-to-severe aphasia (Boyle, 2010). Maddy, Capilouto, and McComas (2012) suggest that SFA is most effective for individuals with fluent aphasia. Additionally, patients must have sufficient cognitive, vision, and hearing abilities to participate in the activity.

Anticipated Outcomes:

The treatment is associated with improvement in naming of trained and untrained nouns. Outcomes measuring related improvements in naming during discourse tasks have been mixed.

To measure outcomes, assess patients using one or more naming tasks. Additionally, gather one or more short discourse samples to assess lexical retrieval in spontaneous speech.

Required Resources:

Graphic organizer, pen, paper, picture of objects

Procedures

SFA treatment is fundamentally a picture naming activity that uses a graphic organizer of semantic features to cue production of the target words. The clinician systematically facilitates identification of the semantic features of each target while facilitating the patient's ability to say the word and ultimately to independently conduct the analysis.

Stimuli Selection

Assess the patient's ability to name a set of pictures (see below for online sources for pictures). Create a large set of pictures from which you can select a smaller set of treatment targets. Based on the patient's response, create two or three treatment sets by selecting pictures the patient could not name and a smaller set of pictures the patient could name to ensure some level of success (for example, two pictures the patient could not name for every one picture the patient could name).

The number of pictures in the assessment and treatment sets will vary depending on the severity of the naming deficit. Patients exhibiting a milder anomia will need a larger assessment set in order to identify difficult items and will be able to practice a greater variety of items during a treatment session.

When creating a treatment set, consider the semantic and phonological similarity between the target words: the greater the similarity, the greater the difficulty level. Patients with a milder anomia may benefit from the challenge posed by the similarity. Reduce similarity, at least in the first treatment set, for patients with a more moderate aphasia.

SFA Chart

Before beginning treatment, design or select an SFA chart to guide the description of each target word. The features to be identified include: Group, Use, Action, Properties, Location, and Association. A number of versions of an SFA are available in the literature (see the Bibliography for links). SFA charts in English and Spanish are provided with the supplemental materials and are available for download at http://www.recipeSLP.com.

Method (Boyle and Coelho, 1995; Boyle, 2004; Coelho, 2007)

Select the set you will use for the first round of treatment. Use this set for each treatment session until the criterion for mastery is met. Repeat the steps listed below for each picture. Even if the patient names the picture correctly in step one, guide the patient through the process of verbalizing the following features of the target: Group, Use, Action, Properties, Location, and Association.

1. Place the picture in the center of the SFA chart.
2. Ask the patient to name the picture-- "What is this?" (Do not name the picture.).
3. Use a question or sentence completion cue to elicit the first feature, Group: "What category does it belong to?" or
   "It is a type of _____."
4. Reinforce the feature by saying it and writing it on the chart.
5. Repeat for each feature.
6. If the chart is completed and the patient has not named the picture, then say the name and ask the patient to repeat it.
7. Review the features of the target word.

Important Tips

- Complete the chart together, even if the patient names the picture during the process.
- Use only those categories appropriate for the target.
- More than one characteristic can be written in a feature box.
- Elicit the features in the same order: Group, Use, Action, Properties, Location, and Association. However, follow the patient's lead if he/she produces the features out of order.
- If the patient is unable to independently provide a description for a category, then say a feature for the client and write it on the chart.
- Give the patient enough, but not too much, time to try to generate the features independently. The amount of time will vary for each patient.
- Focus on the features that most distinguish the target from other related words (For example, if the target is "lemon" features like yellow and sour distinguish it from a similar fruit like an orange.).
- Some clinicians provide additional cues (such as phonological or written cues) if the patient has not named the word after the chart is completed (for example, see Epperly and Flynn, 2008)
- If the patient provides an incorrect name for the picture, then acknowledge the attempt and encourage him/her to keep working through the features to get to the target name.
- Accept synonyms for the target word as a correct response (for example, soda or pop).
- Present each picture only one time during each session.
- Randomize the order of presentation from session to session.
- Use the same pictures until the patient-specific criterion established for success is met.
- For patients with a mild or moderate anomia make the task more challenging by removing the chart after it is completed and the target named. Ask the patient to state the name and describe the target without reading the chart. Provide cues as needed.
- Over time, the role of the clinician should decrease as the patient takes increasing responsibility for the feature analysis.

SFA in Action

Below is an example of a typical client-clinician exchange during SFA. Note that we skip the action category because in the case of the target word "television" action and use are similar. The client provides no response to the "group" question and is given a second prompt before the clinician provides an answer. In this example, the patient says the word during the SFA review, but the process continues through the remaining categories.

The clinician shows the patient a picture of a television.

Clinician: What is this?

Patient: Uhh, yeah, like to watch.

Clinician: Great. It's something you like to watch. [writes "watch" in USE category]

Clinician: What group does it belong to?

Patient: Uhmmm. [shrugs shoulders and shakes head]

Clinician: It's a type of _____.

Patient: Uhh, radio but more."

Clinician: Right, it's like a radio." [writes "radio" in ASSOCIATES category]

Clinician: I would say this belongs to the group electronics. [writes "electronics" in GROUP category]

Clinician: You said you like to watch it. Is there anything else you use it for?

Patient: Uhh, no, watch, watch shows and stuff.

Clinician: [writes "shows" next to "watch"] Excellent. You use it to watch shows.

Clinician: What is it like?

8

Patient: Well.. it's like a.. like a… television…television!

Clinician: That's great! It's a television. You got it. Let's keep describing it. What's it like?

Patient: Uhh, it's a television… some big, some little.

Clinician: It comes in different sizes. It can be big or little. [writes "big or little" in the PROPERTIES box]

Clinician: What else is it like?

Patient: TV is [makes shape of a rectangular with hands].

Clinician: It's shaped like a rectangle, and it can be big or small. Excellent. [writes "rectangle" in PROPERTIES box]

Clinician: Where do you find it?

Patient: Uhmm, me lots of places… couch room.

Clinician: The room with the couch? You find it in the living room?

Patient: Yes, living room and bedroom.

Clinician: True, you find it in the living room and the bedroom.

Patient: And at gym.

Clinician: Good point. You find it in the living room, bedroom, and the gym. [writes each word in the LOCATION box]

Clinician: And, you've already said it's like a radio.

Clinician: [pointing to each box in turn]. So you said it's a type of electronics that you use to watch shows. It can be big or small but is usually rectangular. You can find it in the living room, bedroom, or gym. And, it's like a radio.

Clinician: [pointing to picture] What is this?

Patient: Uhh, te- tev- television.

Clinician: Great! It's a television. Ready for the next one?

Online Sources for Pictures

Once you have created the larger set of pictures, it can be used with different patients. A number of websites provide free access to picture stimuli that can be downloaded and printed.

- The International Picture Naming Project offers 244 publically available object pictures. http://crl.ucsd.edu/experiments/ipnp/method/getpics/getpics.html
- The Amsterdam Library of Object Images offers hundreds of color pictures for download. http://aloi.science.uva.nl/
- Bonin et al., have made available a set of 299 black-and-white line drawings. http://leadserv.u-bourgogne.fr/bases/pictures/

Variations and Modifications

Elaborated Semantic Feature Analysis (Papathanasiou, Mesolora, Mihou, and Papachristou, 2006)

Complete SFA as described in the previous chapter. After the chart is completed and the picture is named, encourage the patient to use the features and target word to form sentences.

Use of SFA in Small Groups (Antonucci, 2009; Falconer and Antonucci, 2012)

The first step in group SFA is to introduce the concept of SFA to group members. Start by completing the SFA process described above with one patient with one target object. After the SFA process is completed, the group discusses if the description was sufficient and if they could recognize the item from the information provided.

Once the patients are familiar with the concept of SFA, future sessions are dedicated to practicing SFA in connected speech using a modified-PACE (Promoting Aphasic Communicative Effectiveness) procedure. Present a picture to one patient so that the other group members cannot see it. He/she then attempts to name or describe the picture for the other members using SFA categories. Encourage the listeners to ask questions and request clarification. Complete the SFA chart even if the speaker or listeners provide the name of the target. After the SFA process is completed, give the listeners a choice of three or four pictures from which to choose the one they believe was the target. Group members take turns being the listeners and the speaker.

SFA Combined with Response Elaboration Training (Conley and Coelho, 2003)

Response Elaboration Training (RET) is a loose training technique that combines a patient's response to two questions to form a more complex response (See RecipeSLP's *The SLP's Guide to Response Elaboration Training* for more information.).

In SFA+RET, follow the SFA procedure as described above. During the naming of the semantic features, ask questions to elicit multiple responses to a category. Chain together two or more responses the patient produced during the SFA procedure to form a more complex response. Model the elaborated response, and ask the patient to repeat it.

For example, present the picture of a dog and ask "What is this?"
Patient: Woof.

SLP: That's right. It makes the sound "woof." Where does it make this sound?

Patient: My house.

SLP: Great. Dog woofs in house. You say that.

Patient: Dog woofs in house.

SLP: Excellent. What does the dog remind you of?

SFA and Discourse Production (Peach and Reuter, 2010)

In this application of SFA, begin by asking the patient to describe a set of pictures depicting a scene and/or ask him/her to describe procedures. Review the patient's responses and generate a list words that he/she was unable to retrieve to use as treatment targets.

1. Start with the first target word.
2. Present the pictures and/or procedures on which the anomia occurred during the probe described above.
3. Bring the target to the patient's attention without naming the target and ask the patient to name the target.
4. If the patient does or does not name the target complete the SFA process as described in the previous chapter.

The SFA procedure includes the following modifications:

- The center of the SFA chart has a blank box for the target word rather than the picture.
- The same picture stimuli and target words are used from session to session, but the order of presentation varies until the criterion established for mastery is met.
- A small number of items (3-4) are trained per session.
- Remaining items are sent home for homework with each target written in the center of a separate chart.

SFA and Contextual Discourse (Rider, Wright, Marshall, and Page, 2008)

The authors paired SFA targets with story retell (using clips from episodes of TV shows such as *Bewitched* and *The Cosby Show*) and procedural discourse (for example, "Tell me how you make a sandwich."). Treatment begins with a probe of the number of words the patient produces for each stimulus (eight clips and/or procedures). Based on the patient's responses a list of 10 words that were and were not produced by the patient is created for each stimulus. Target words should be highly salient for the specific context. Train each list one at a time following the SFA procedures describe in the previous chapter. The authors set a criterion for mastery of a set at a maximum ten sessions or 80% of words on the list correct across two sessions. After a list has been mastered, re-probe response to the corresponding clip or procedure.

Covert SFA (Coppens and Mylott, 2006)

This SFA method reduces the time required to complete each SFA without sacrificing accuracy, particularly for patients whose expressive language is labored. Once the patient understands and practices traditional SFA, introduce the concept of covert SFA, which involves thinking about the features rather than saying them aloud.

1. Instruct the patient to concentrate and think about the feature.
2. Tell the patient to indicate (verbally or non-verbally) when he/she is ready to move on to the next feature.
3. Encourage the patient to name the target at any point in the process.
4. After the patient has indicated he/she has reviewed all the features, prompt him/her to name the picture.
5. If the patient is unable to name the word, review the features aloud using single words and short phrases and ask the patient to repeat each feature.
6. Ask the patient to name the picture.
7. If the patient does not name the picture, then provide a phonemic cue.
8. If the patient does not name the picture, then provide the word and ask the patient to repeat it.

SFA and Story Retell (Insalaco, Gugino, and Ulicki, 2007)

SFA story re-tell treatment involves creating stories in which target words are embedded along with 2 or more features for each word.

1. Present the picture of each target word for the patient to name.
2. Complete SFA for any pictures not named.
3. Read the story as the pictures are shown again.
4. Instruct the patient to repeat the target word and the features.
5. Re-tell the story.
6. Instruct the patient to re-tell the story and encourage him/her to point to the pictures.

SFA with Personally Relevant Features (Carvey-Essenburg, Patterson, and Avent, J., 2006)

This modified SFA treatment encourages a patient to describe targets using personally relevant features. This treatment uses color pictures for the following procedure.

1. Present the patient with a set of pictures and ask him/her to select a relevant noun.
2. Discuss the semantic features of the target.
3. Write the cues on the back of the picture.
4. Ask the patient to choose the "best" cue. (This cue will be the first one presented in subsequent sessions.)
5. Read the "best" cue.
6. Ask the patient to repeat the "best" cue.
7. Ask the patient to name the target.
8. Repeat to each additional target word.

Naming TherAppy

Naming TherAppy by Tactus is an iPad app designed around the concept of Semantic Feature Analysis, though it deviates in significant ways from the procedures described above (http://tactustherapy.com/apps/naming/).

The vocabulary options include over 500 nouns, 100 verbs, 100 adjectives, and unlimited custom photos. Four modes are built into the app: naming practice, description, test, and personalized flash cards. A six-step hierarchy includes both semantic and phonological cues.

A number of reviews for Naming TherAppy are available online.
http://ispeakapp.com/2011/08/30/naming-therappy/
http://slpecho.wordpress.com/2013/02/19/naming-therappy-a-review/

NameThat!

Name That! is an iPad and Android app designed to help people with aphasia improve naming and describing abilities. Developed by speech-language pathologists at the University of Iowa, the app includes 130 pictures across 12 semantic categories. While the app is described as having a basis in Semantic Feature Analysis, it differs from SFA in a number of significant ways. It does not use a multiple features to describe each target nor does it guide the user through these features. Rather, it provides a written semantic question which the user must answer with no feedback or support. The user can then select one or both phonological cues (initial syllable or whole word) to hear and see the target word. It is unclear from the app description if this app is intended to be done with the SLP present. Given the format, an SLP or trained caregiver would need to be working with the patient to provide feedback on the identification of sematic features. Additionally, the patient must have the ability read the question prompt (e.g. "How would you describe this?") as there is no audio for the prompt.

Additional information can be found at: http://www.jpec.org/AppsLab/NameThat

A Summary of the Theory and Evidence

The EBP Triangle

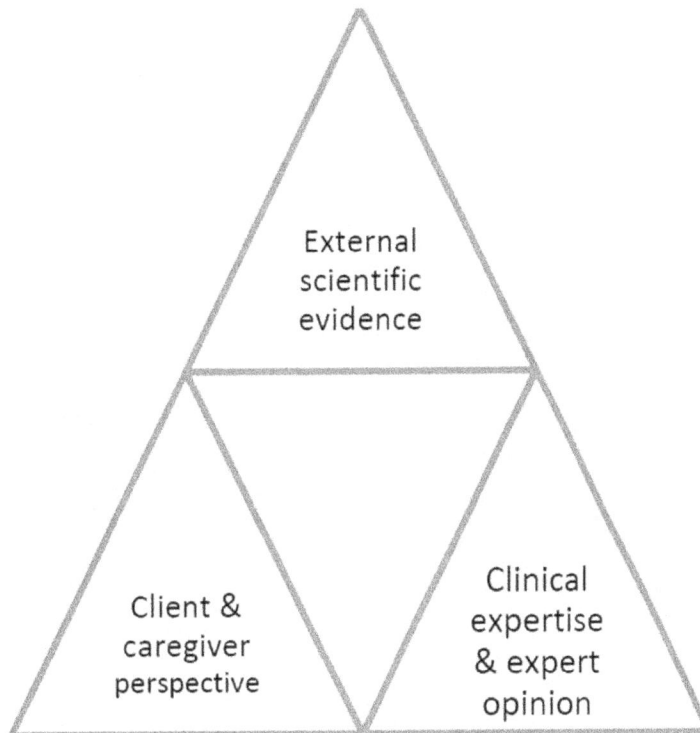

Theory

SFA is based on the theory that normal lexical access results from the simultaneous activation of features that sum together to trigger the selection of a target response. Some features include the characteristics of the target, variations of the target, semantically related words, and phonologically related words. For example,

- Target: dog
- Production of "dog" results from activation of concepts such as fur, pet, puppy, cat, house, hog, four-legged, animal, and/or bark.

SFA restores semantic access by strengthening the activation of the semantic features in order to trigger the production of the target word.

External Scientific Evidence

Mary Boyle (2010) provides a thorough overview of SFA and supporting evidence. She reports on seven published studies that measured outcomes of SFA (in its various forms) used with participants with aphasia. Overall, the participants of these studies demonstrated improved naming on trained stimuli. However, results measuring generalization and maintenance of improvement over time were mixed. Since 2010, six additional single subject studies reporting positive outcomes from the use of SFA for participants with aphasia have been published.

Maddy, Capilouto and McComas (2012) conducted a systematic review of published research into SFA. Their analysis includes seven single subject studies involving sixteen participants in total. Results suggest that SFA was most effective for individuals with fluent aphasia. Some patients did not appear to benefit from SFA.

Evidence for the variations and modifications of SFA described in the previous chapter are generally limited to one or two studies utilizing single subject or case series designs. Generally, studies report improvement on picture naming for trained words. Generalization to untrained words and discourse varies. Generalization to discourse appears to be better for those studies that actively incorporate a discourse element during the treatment procedure (such as group SFA).

No data were found supporting the specific effectiveness of Naming TherAppy and Name That!, Both deviate from SFA in that they provide phonological cues. Of the two, Naming TherAppy is most consistent with SFA as it has been described in the existing research. Name That! uses few of the elements that typify SFA, particularly the use of a graphic organizer and the review of multiple semantic features. Given the structure of Name That! it is likely that patients using the app independently would rely more heavily on the phonological cues; stimulation of the semantic system would be limited.

A search of the Clinical Aphasiology Conference proceedings resulted in 19 unique studies that referenced SFA.

(http://aphasiology.pitt.edu/),

a number of which were later published.

The American Speech-Language-Hearing Association (ASHA) Practice Portal for aphasia states that the evidence supports the use of phonological and semantic cueing strategies to improve naming accuracy.

http://www.asha.org/PRPSpecificTopic.aspx?folderid=8589934663&section=Treatment

The ASHA Evidence Map for aphasia states that the evidence indicates semantic, phonological, and mixed cuing strategies are efficacious.

http://www.ncepmaps.org/Aphasia-Treatment-Word-Finding.php

The Academy of Neurologic Communication Disorders and Sciences (ANCDS) developed evidence tables for studies on lexical retrieval, including SFA.

http://aphasiatx.arizona.edu/lexical

Clinical Expertise and Expert Opinion

Clinical interest in the use of SFA with aphasia is substantial. A search for "semantic feature analysis aphasia" on the ASHA website (1/24/2014) produced 100 results. SFA has been mentioned in 54 ASHA convention presentations, 10 journal articles, and 9 ASHA Leader articles.

The finding that better SFA outcomes are associated with fluent aphasia is consistent with the semantic nature of both the treatment and naming deficits associated with fluent aphasia. Clinicians should use naming assessments and error analysis to characterize the semantic and/or phonological nature of the patient's anomia in order to determine the appropriateness of SFA for a particular patient. The lack of generalization to discourse should be considered in treatment planning. Clinicians may choose to incorporate procedures that support the use of the treatment targets in connected speech.

Patient and caregiver perspective

Boyle and Coehlo (1995) report that improvement in naming following SFA was associated with improvement on the Communicative Effectiveness Inventory (a rating scale measuring a patient's perception of his/her functional communication). Clinical experience suggests that patients vary greatly in their ability to independently generate the semantic features. Given practice, they begin to understand the SFA process and enjoy the challenge posed by the SFA chart.

References

Antonucci, S. M. (2009). Use of semantic feature analysis in group aphasia treatment. *Aphasiology, 23*(7-8), 854-866.

Boyle, M. (2004). Semantic feature analysis treatment for anomia in two fluent aphasia syndromes. *American Journal of Speech-Language Pathology*, 13(3), 236-249. http://ajslp.pubs.asha.org/article.aspx?articleid=1774785

Boyle, M. (2010). Semantic feature analysis treatment for aphasic word retrieval impairments: what's in a name? *Topics in Stroke Rehabilitation, 17*(6), 411-422.

Boyle, M., & Coelho, C. A. (1995). Application of semantic feature analysis as a treatment for aphasic dysnomia. *American Journal of Speech-Language Pathology, 4,* 94-98. http://ajslp.pubs.asha.org/article.aspx?articleid=1774521

Carvey-Essenburg, H., Patterson, J., & Avent, J. (2006). Personalized semantic cuing treatment for naming deficit in a person with conduction aphasia. Paper presented at the American Speech Language and Hearing Convention, Miami, FL. www.asha.org/Events/convention/handouts/2006/1800_Carvey-Essenburg_Hannah/

Coelho, C. A., McHugh, R. E., & Boyle, M. (2000). Semantic feature analysis as a treatment for aphasic dysnomia: A replication. *Aphasiology, 14*(2), 133-142.

Coppens, P., & Mylott, A. (2006). Covert semantic feature analysis therapy for severe broca aphasia. American Speech Language and Hearing Convention, Miami, FL. www.asha.org/Events/convention/handouts/2010/2183-Pernacchio-Amy/

Epperly, R., & Flynn, J. (2008). The use of semantic feature analysis with wernicke's aphasia. American Speech Language and Hearing Convention, Chicago, IL. www.asha.org/Events/convention/handouts/2008/2267_Epperly_Rebecca/

Falconer, C., & Antonucci, S. M. (2012). Use of semantic feature analysis in group discourse treatment for aphasia: Extension and expansion. *Aphasiology, 26*(1), 64-82.

Hashimoto, N., & Frome, A. (2011). The use of a modified semantic features analysis approach in aphasia. *Journal of Communication Disorders, 44*(4), 459-469.

Hough, M. and King, K. (2008). Enhancing Word Retrieval in Three Adults With Chronic Fluent Aphasia. Clinical Aphasiology Conference. http://aphasiology.pitt.edu/archive/00001931/01/viewpaper.pdf

Insalaco, D., Gugino, C., & Ulicki, M. (2007). Semantic feature analysis treatment as a bridge to narrative. Paper presented at American Speech Language and Hearing Convention, Boston, MA. www.asha.org/Events/convention/handouts/2007/1101_Insalaco_Deborah/

Maddy, K., Capilouto, G. and McComas, K. (2012). The efficacy of semantic feature analysis for the treatment of aphasia: A systematic review. Clinical Aphasiology Conference. http://aphasiology.pitt.edu/archive/00002378/01/227-367-1-RV_%28Maddy_Capilouto_McComas%29.pdf

Muñoz, M.L. (2014). *The method and science of Reducing Aphasic Perseveration*. Recipe SLP, Fort Worth, TX.

Peach, R. K., & Reuter, K. A. (2010). A discourse-based approach to semantic feature analysis for the treatment of aphasic word retrieval failures. *Aphasiology, 24*(9), 971-990.

Papathanasiou, I., Mesolora, A., Mihou, E., and Papachristou, G. (2006). Elaborated semantic feature analysis treatment: Lexicality and generalization effects in a case with anomic aphasia. Clinical Aphasiology Conference. http://aphasiology.pitt.edu/archive/00002180/01/264.pdf

Rider, J. D., Wright, H. H., Marshall, R. C., & Page, J. L. (2008). Using semantic feature analysis to improve contextual discourse in adults with aphasia. *American Journal of Speech-Language Pathology, 17*(2), 161-172. http://ajslp.pubs.asha.org/article.aspx?articleid=1757568

van Hees, S., Angwin, A., McMahon, K., & Copland, D. (2013). A comparison of semantic feature analysis and phonological components analysis for the treatment of naming impairments in aphasia. *Neuropsychological Rehabilitation, 23*(1), 102-132.

II - RESPONSE ELABORATION TRAINING (RET)

Response Elaboration Training (RET)

Purpose:

RET uses a loose-training technique to improve a patients' ability to increase the production of content words in spontaneous speech in order to "more fully share the burden of communication with [his/her] partners" (Kearns and Scher, 1985, p. 224). The patient initiates a series of prompted responses to a stimulus. These responses combine to form a single response containing more content words.

Intended Population:

RET has been used successfully with patients exhibiting a variety of aphasia types and severities. However, maintenance and generalization of increased verbal output appear to be poorer for individuals with fluent aphasia (Wambaugh, Wright, and Nessler, 2012). Modified RET (mRET) was developed for patients with both aphasia and moderate to severe apraxia.

Anticipated Outcomes:

The treatment is designed to increase the number of content words in a patient's utterances. Pre- and post-treatment, the number of content words, and particularly context appropriate words, should be measured on one or more discourse tasks, such as: picture description, procedural discourse, personal narratives, and/or conversation.

Required Resources:

Stimuli (action pictures or procedural prompts), pen, paper, and response tracking sheet (available at http://www.recipeslp.com).

Getting Ready for RET and Modified RET

RET involves the use of a picture description activity during which the clinician systematically facilitates the expansion of patient-initiated verbal responses using Wh- questions within a forward chaining technique. The purpose of RET is to systematically increase the number of content words and the length of utterance in the spontaneous speech of individuals with aphasia (Wambaugh, et al., 2012).

Stimuli

Before beginning RET, create 1 or more sets of 10 pictures to use in training. The number of pictures in a set can be adjusted based on the severity of the patient's aphasia and the length of the treatment session. Use the same set of pictures until an established criterion for mastery is met.

RET requires the use of drawings or photos that depict a clear action. Research has used primarily action pictures that have few details other than the subject and the action in order to encourage the generation of a more imaginative response (Kearns and Scher, 1988). However, clinicians may need to use functional or readily available pictures depicting actions in more complex contexts.

Wambaugh and Martinez (2000) include a list of the action scenes depicted in each set of experimental pictures. Actions included playing, tying, opening, reading, hanging, throwing, blowing, cleaning, licking, writing, cutting, drinking, and locking. Bennett, et al. (2006) include a list of 36 verbs depicted in their experimental stimuli.

Drawings and photos can be obtained from a variety of sources such as Google Images. A set of 129 black and white line-drawings depicting a variety of actions can be downloaded for free from the International Picture Naming Project (IPNP) website at http://crl.ucsd.edu/experiments/ipnp/actobj/getpics/getpics.html.

Measuring Outcomes

The effect of RET on spoken language has been measured as the number of content words the client produces spontaneously in response to the picture (Kearns and Scher, 1988). Content words include nouns, pronouns, main verbs, adjectives, adverbs, and prepositions. To be counted, the word must relate to the picture in some way but does not actually have to be depicted in picture.

Research on mRET has used calculations of correct information units (CIUs) to measure outcomes (Wambaugh and Martinez, 2000). Nicholas and Brookshire (1993) introduced CIUs as a way to measure the effectiveness and efficiency of connected speech. Determining if a word is a CIU in mRET involves more complicated decision making than measuring content words due to the acceptable variability in patient responses. A link to the original study by Nicholas and Brookshire (1993) is provided in the bibliography for readers who want to further explore the defining criteria for CIUs. However, this review of RET will focus on measuring progress based on an increase in the number of content words.

Before beginning treatment on any picture set, conduct a probe to determine the average number of content words produced by the patient. For each picture in the set, provide the client with a prompt such as, "Tell me as much as you can about this picture or anything that it reminds you of." Count the number of content words in each response and then calculate the average number of words in a response for the set (total number of content words divided by number of pictures). The criterion for mastery then is set at a number greater than the average calculated during the probe. The clinician can establish a criterion for mastery of a set based on one or more of the following measures (with examples):

- the average number of content words (the average is 2.75, so a criterion of 3.75 is set, corresponding with one additional word),

- the range or responses (the range is 2-4 so a criterion is set at 4-6 words on 80% of responses), or

- the best response (the patient's best response is 4 words but the average is 2.5, so a criterion of an average of 4 words is set).

During treatment, the number of content words is taken from the patient's initial response to the picture before the initial elaboration question is asked (Step 2 in the next chapter). A set is trained until the criterion for mastery is met. The next treatment set should be probed to establish the best criteria for that set.

Picture Prompts

One of a number of prompts can be used to elicit the patient's initial response (Step 2 in the next chapter), including the following (Kearns and Scher, 1988; Wambaugh, Wright, and Nessler, 2012):

- Tell me as much as you can about this picture or anything that it reminds you of.

- Tell me about this picture.

- What does this remind you of?

- Tell me what's happening.

Elaboration is solicited using one Wh- question (*who, what, where, when, why, or how*). Without expecting a specific response, consider selecting Wh- questions that encourage production of the most meaningful elements in the picture.

RET Procedures

RET Method (Kearns, 1985; Kearns and Scher, 1988; Gaddie, Kearns, and Yoder, 1989)

The key to RET is following the patient's lead. The pictures provide a context for building the response, but no specific response is expected. Use Wh- questions to systematically expand the patient's expression of his/her perspective or opinion.

The basic structure of the treatment is described below. A sample exchange is provided in a following section to illustrate the clinician-client interaction.

1. Present the target picture.

2. Instruct the patient to "tell me as much as you can about this picture or anything that it reminds you of."

    2.1. Patient responds. [count content words in this response to measure progress]

3. Repeat an expanded form of the client's response and reinforce it.

4. Ask a Wh- question.

    4.1. Patient responds.

5. Say an elaborated response by combining the meaningful elements of the patient's two responses.

6. 6 Tell the patient "Repeat after me" and restate the elaborated response.

    6.1. Patient repeats.

7. Reinforce the model.

8. 8 Elicit a delayed repetition of the elaborated response.

    8.1. Patient repeats.

9. Repeat steps 4-8 until the patient is unable to repeat the elaborated response. [Optional Step].

10. Present the next picture in the set.

Important Tips for RET

- Gaddie et al. (1989) provide a flowchart of the RET process. The chart includes guidance for clinicians regarding how they should react to certain types of client responses. A number of these points are described in this section.

- The clinician may follow the RET process with the same picture multiple times (Step 9) or just once (skip Step 9 and go to Step 10).

- Remember that RET is built around a patient initiated response. Spontaneous speech is the building block for the more elaborated response, so follow the patient's lead. The patient's response is valued for its communicative intent.

- If the patient is unable to repeat the elaborated response, then move on to the next item.

- Though no specific response is being targeted, the words should relate to the picture in some way.

- Irrelevant responses, unrelated responses, and lack of response should be managed in a similar manner. If the patient does not respond or provides an unrelated response to an initial or Wh- question prompt, then repeat the prompt (or a similar prompt). If the patient still does not respond or provides an irrelevant response, then move on to the next picture.

- If the patient has persistent difficulties formulating a response, then consider using mRET to implement different prompting procedures.

- If the patient's response is incompatible with the Wh- question asked (e.g. the patient provides *what* information to a *why* question), then repeat and reinforce an elaborated response using the patient's response. Ask the Wh- question that matches the patient's response so that he/she can repeat the response in the context of the matching question. Continue with the next step in the RET process.

- Consider the complexity of the sentence that is likely to result from a particular question in relation to the client's level of severity. A client who is saying one word is unlikely to be able to produce a sentence elaborated by a "Why" question since the response will generally require complex syntax.

- Model a response that is consistent to the number of words established as the criteria for mastery.

- Be clear on the length of response modeled for and expected from the client. A patient producing single words might be expected to expand to a 2-4 word response. A patient producing 3-4 word phrases may be expected to expand to 5-7 word responses.

- The phrases modeled by the clinician may or may not be syntactically complete. For example, when expanding to three words, the response may be "The man sits" (syntactic) or "Man hits ball" (missing functor words), depending on the responses provided by the patient.

- The elaborated response modeled by the clinician must be semantically plausible.

RET in Action

Below are two examples of exchanges that could result from the same picture. In Version 2, the clinician provided additional prompts and modeling to facilitate production of the elaborated response. Additionally, the elaboration with a Wh- question is conducted twice until the patient cannot repeat the elaborated sentence accurately. The patient should produce the phrase or sentence as the clinician stated it. The focus is on helping the patient to produce a response that has more words than the patient's initial response.

Version 1: [Clinician presents a picture of a woman riding a bike.]

Clinician: Tell me as much as you can about this picture or anything that it reminds you of.

Patient: Uhh, woman, umm, bike... Yeah... woman, bike, and uhmm....

Clinician: Excellent. The woman is on a bike.

Clinician: What is the woman doing on the bike?

Patient: Uhh woman... riding... umm... bike...uhh riding bike.

Clinician: Great. The woman is riding a bike.

Clinician: Now, you say it. The woman is riding a bike.

Patient: The woman...is riding the...bike.

Clinician: Excellent. The woman is riding a bike.

Clinician: Great. Now, I'm going to show you the picture, and I want you to repeat what you just said about the picture. [points to picture]. What is happening in this picture?

Patient: The woman...is riding...the bike.

Clinician: Excellent. The woman is riding a bike. Ready for the next picture?

Version 2: [Clinician presents a picture of a woman riding a bike.]

Clinician: Tell me as much as you can about this picture or anything that it reminds you of.

Patient: Uhh, yeah, yeah....

Clinician: Tell me what's happening.

Patient: Woman going.

Clinician: Great. Where is the woman going?

Patient: Bike.

Clinician: Ok. What is the woman riding?

Patient: Bike.

Clinician: Great. The woman is riding a bike. You say it. The woman is riding a bike.

Patient: Uhhh... woman... bike...

Clinician: Try it again. The woman is riding the bike.

Patient: The woman is riding the bike.

Clinician: Excellent. The woman is riding the bike. Now, I'm going to show you the picture, and I want you to repeat the sentence.

Clinician: [points to picture] Tell me about this picture.

Patient: The woman is riding the bike

Clinician: Great. The woman is riding the bike. Where is the woman going?

Patient: Going?

Clinician: Yes. Where is the woman going?

Patient: Uhmm, maybe the woman going to uhh store.

Clinician: That's possible. The woman is going to the store. The woman on the bike is going to the store.

Clinician: Now, you say it. The woman on the bike is going to the store.

Patient: The woman... bike...uhh... is going store.

Clinician: Close. Listen again. The woman on the bike is going to the store.

Patient: The woman on bike...uhh...is going store.

Clinician: Better. The woman on the bike is going to the store. Why don't we go on to the next picture? Ready?

Modified RET Procedures

mRET (Wambaugh and Martinez, 2000; Wambaugh, 2007; Wambaugh, Wright, and Nessler, 2012)

mRET maintains the purpose of RET but provides additional support for individuals with both aphasia and moderate to severe apraxia. Developed by Julie Wambaugh and colleagues, mRET incorporates strategies known to facilitate improvement in speech production (such as repeated practice and integral stimulation) with standard RET procedures (Wambaugh and Martinez, 2000). mRET incorporates additional opportunities for clinician modeling, practice, integral stimulation, and time delayed response. For additional information, readers are directed to Wambaugh, Wright, and Nessler (2012), who provide a detailed step-by-step guide for conducting mRET.

Present the target picture.

1. Instruct the patient to "Tell me about this picture."

    1.1 Evaluate the patient's response.If correct (e.g. is understood and relates to the picture), then move to Step 3.

    1.2 If incorrect or no response, implement cueing hierarchy (see steps below).

2. Say and reinforce the client's response.

3. Ask a Wh- question.

4. Evaluate the patient's response.

    4.1 If correct, then move to Step 6.

    4.2 If incorrect or no response, implement cueing hierarchy (see steps below).

5. Reinforce the correct response and model an expanded response by combining the meaning elements of the patient's two responses (Steps 3 and 6).

6. Tell the patient "Repeat after me." Then, restate the expanded response.

7. Evaluate the patient's response.

    7.1 If correct, ask client to repeat the response three times.

    7.2 If incorrect, attempt to elicit up to four productions of the target using integral stimulation (see steps below).

8. Remove the picture and wait at least five seconds.

9. Present the picture again and ask the patient to describe the picture.

    9.1 If the patient produces the ENTIRE response, then reinforce the production.

    9.2 If the patient provides an incomplete response or no response, then model the response and request a production with integral stimulation.

    9.3 If an alternate correct response is produced, then reinforce the response.

10. Repeat the process for each remaining picture.

Cueing Hierarchy

If the patient provides an incorrect response or fails to respond at Steps 2 or 5, implement the following cueing hierarchy.

Give two possible response options ("You can say something like X [noun phrase] or Y [verb phrase].").

1 If the patient repeats one of the choices, then move to the next step in the mRET process.

2 If the patient provides an incorrect response or no response, then model a one word response (noun or verb) and ask the patient to "Say ___."

2.1 If the patient is correct, move to the next step in the mRET process.

2.2 If the patient is incorrect or produces no response, then use integral stimulation (see steps below) to elicit a noun or verb. Give up to 4 attempts for the patient to produce a correct response.

2.2.a If the patient is correct, move to the next step in the mRET process.

2.2.b If the patient is incorrect after 4 attempts, move to the next item.

Integral Stimulation (Rosenbek and Wertz, 1972; Rosenbek et al., 1973)

Integral Stimulation is an eight step hierarchy for treating acquired apraxia of speech in adults that uses the systematic application of "integral stimulation," which involves the use of visual ("Watch me.") and auditory ("Listen to me.") cues. All eight steps are completed for each target. If the patient has difficulty with the word at one integral stimulation level, then fall back to the previous level. Allow up to 4 attempts to say the word/phrase at each integral stimulation level. If the patient is unable to produce the target after four attempts at one integral stimulation level, then move to the next picture in the mRET training set.

1. Tell the patient to "Watch me" and "Listen to me." Say the word. The clinician and the patient then say the word together.
2. Tell the patient to "Watch me" and "Listen to me." Say the word. Then mouth the word silently as the patient says it.
3. Tell the patient to "Watch me" and "Listen to me." Tell the patient "Repeat after me." Say the word and then the patient says it.
4. Tell the patient to "Watch me" and "Listen to me." Say the word once then ask the patient to repeat it multiple times.
5. Present the written word and ask the patient to say it.
6. Present the written word, remove it, and then ask the patient to say it.
7. Ask a question to elicit the response.
8. Use role-play to elicit the target response.

Important Tips

- The tips provided for RET also apply to mRET.

- When integral stimulation is needed, the clinician should start with Step 1 and proceed through each step as described. The steps for integral stimulation should be conducted in order, but steps can be skipped as appropriate for the particular client. In particular, Steps 7 and 8 may be difficult to complete when working at the single word level.

- During integral stimulation, placement and motoric cues can be provided as needed.

- Integral stimulation allows for minor omissions, distortions, or substitutions that do not impact the meaning of the message.

mRET in Action

Below are two examples of exchanges that could result from the same picture. In Version 2, the patient produces apraxic errors that require more modeling and the use of integral stimulation. Notice that Step 8 of integral stimulation is skipped since the client is working at the single word level. For clarity, the integral stimulation steps are identified in brackets, e.g. [1].

Version 1: [Clinician presents a picture of a woman riding a bike.]

Clinician: Tell me about this picture.

Patient: Uhh…. Man… no… uhm… man… no….

Clinician: You can say something like "young woman" or "riding a bike."

Patient: Uhh…the man… no!

Clinician: Say "woman."

Patient: Uhh th… wo… woman…woman.

Clinician: Great. Woman. That is a woman.

Clinician: What is the woman doing?

Patient: Uhh buh buh bike! Bike!

Clinician: Excellent. "Woman rides bike."

Clinician: Now, you say it. "Woman rides bike."

Patient: Woman rides bike.

Clinician: Great. Now, say it two more times.

Patient: Woman rides bike.

Patient: Woman rides bike.

[Clinician removes picture and waits 5 seconds.]

Clinician: Tell me as much as you can about this picture.

Patient: Woman… rides… bike.

Clinician: Nice! Woman rides bike.

Clinician: Are you ready for the next one?

Version 2: [Clinician presents a picture of a woman riding a bike.]

Clinician: Tell me as much as you can about this picture or anything that it reminds you of.

Patient: Uhh…. Man… no… uhm… man… no….

Clinician: You can say something like "young woman" or "rides bike."

Patient: Uhh…the man… no!

Clinician: Say "woman."

Patient: Uhh th… wo… wodan…wodan.

Clinician: Close. Watch me and listen carefully. Woman. Now, say it with me. [1]

Client and Clinician: Woman.

Clinician: Now, watch me and say the word "woman." [2]

Client: Woman [as clinician mouths the word].

Clinician: Now, I'll say it, then you say it. Woman. [3]

Client: Woman.

Clinician: Excellent. Now, say woman five times. Watch me. "Woman." [4]

Client: Woman. Woman. Woman. Woman. Woman.

Clinician: Great.

[Clinician writes "woman" and shows it to the client.]

Clinician: Read this word. [5]

Clinician/Client: "Woman."

[Present the paper with the word written on it, then remove it.]

Clinician: What word did you read? [6]

Client: Woman.

Clinician: Who is in the picture? [7]

Client: Woman.

Clinician: Excellent. Now, what is the woman doing?

Patient: Uhh buh buh bike! Bike!

Clinician: Excellent. Woman rides bike.

Clinician: Now, you say it. The woman rides bike.

Patient: Woman.. .uhh…bike.

Clinician: Close. Listen and watch. "Woman rides bike."

Clinician: Now, say it with me, "Woman rides bike."

Patient: Bike uhhh wide, uh no.

Clinician: Listen and watch. "Woman rides bike."

Clinician: Now say it with me, "Woman rides bike."

Patient: Uhh woman… and uhh… blike.

Clinician: Listen and watch. "Woman rides bike."

Clinician: Now, say it with me, "Woman rides bike."

Patient: Wodan no wodan wondan…dang it.

Clinician: Let's try it one more time. Listen and watch. "Woman rides bike."

Clinician: Now, say it with me, "Woman rides bike."

Patient: Wodan…. Woman.. blike…bike… uhhh. Uhh.

Clinician: You're getting closer. Let's move on to the next. Are you ready?

Variations

A number of studies report variations of the use of RET and mRET. In their research on mRET, Wambaugh and colleagues studied the implementation of mRET with picture description, personal recounts, and procedure prompts. Variation in elicitation procedures was done in part to examine the extent to which increase in CIU's generalized to discourse. Conley and Coelho (2003) report on the use of RET as a supplemental procedure for Semantic Feature Analysis as a way to further strengthen the activation and retrieval of the target words.

Procedural Discourse (Wambaugh et al., 2012 and 2013)

The initial prompt is "Tell me in detail how you...." for common procedures. A full list of 20 procedures is provided by Wambaugh et al., (2012 and 2013). Procedures should be familiar to the patient and allow for variations related to personal and cultural preferences. Procedures might include such activities as moving to a new house, getting groceries, making a sandwich, scrambling eggs, doing laundry, changing a tire, getting ready to go on vacation, going to the dentist, planning a birthday party, or going to a movie.

The steps are similar to those previously described for mRET with some minor modifications. When providing a model for the patient, the clinician's focus is on modeling procedural steps rather than a noun phrase and/or verb phrase. Elaborated responses are specific to the procedure. Finally, the clinician requires the patient to re-tell the complete procedure to the best of his/her abilities.

Personal Recounts (Wambaugh, et al., 2013)

Wambaugh and colleagues studied the use of personal recounts as the stimulus for mRET. For personal recounts, the clinician asks the patient to "tell me something about anything that you would like to talk about." The results for use of personal recounts have been extremely mixed, and this procedure is not recommended at this time.

SFA Combined with Response Elaboration Training (Conley and Coelho, 2003)

Semantic Feature Analysis (SFA) is a technique that facilitates naming using a graphic organizer to elicit features of the target (see RecipeSLP's *The SLP's Guide to Semantic Feature Analysis* for more information). In SFA+RET, the SFA procedures are the guiding elements and RET is embedded to encourage generalization of naming success to connected speech.

During the naming of the semantic features, ask questions to elicit multiple responses to a category. Chain together two or more responses the patient produced during the SFA procedure to form a more complex response. Model the elaborated response and ask the patient to repeat it.

For example, present the picture of a dog and ask, "What is this?"

Patient: Woof.

SLP: That's right. It makes the sound "woof." Where does it make this sound?

Patient: My house.

SLP: Great. The dog woofs in your house. You say that.

Patient: Dog woofs in house.

SLP: Excellent. What does the dog remind you of?

Notice that while the patient's repetition does not exactly match the model, it is a more complex response than what he/she produced spontaneously.

A Summary of the Theory and Evidence

The EBP Triangle

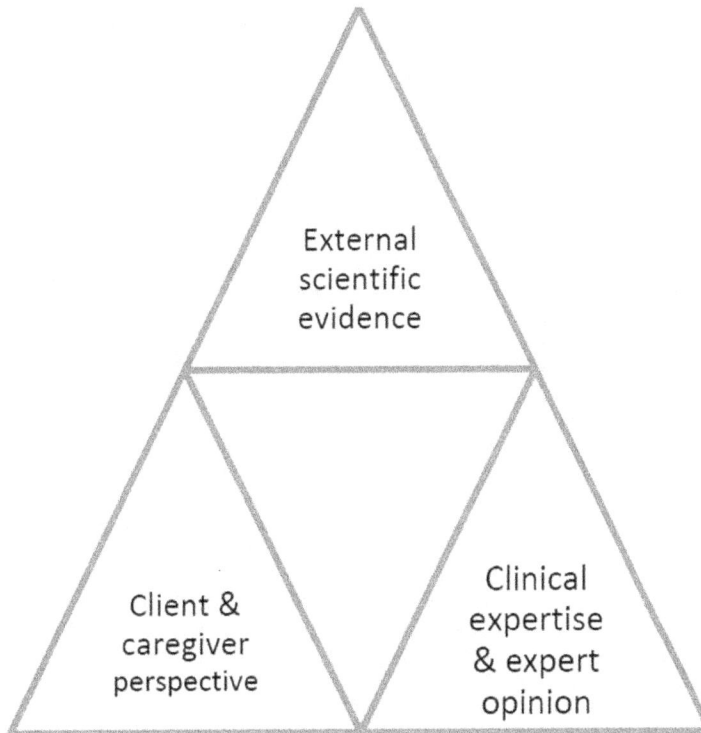

Theory

RET was initially developed based on Hart and Risley's Incidental Teaching approach to child language intervention, which supports ideas of patient-initiated responses, naturalistic feedback, and a focus on content over form (Kearns, 1985). RET is a "loose training" approach that emphasizes response flexibility and the shaping of patient initiated responses. RET focuses on pragmatic and communicative aspects of language by emphasizing content over form. Additionally, it puts the burden of communication on the patient rather than the clinician.

RET is based on the belief that didactic training inhibits creativity and flexible language use and has limited generalization (Kearns and Scher, 1988). Loose training reduces clinician control over stimulus, response, and feedback and facilitates improvement in generalized responding by increasing the range of stimulus conditions and response options compared to what is typically seen in didactic treatment (Gaddie et al., 1989). Additionally, RET incorporates aspects of cognitive stimulation by requiring fluency, flexibility, originality, elaboration, and divergent thinking (Chapey, 2008).

RET can be considered an error-reduced procedure (Chapey, 2008). The forward chaining technique allows for the systematic and incremental increase in the number of content units in a patient's verbal response.

Wambaugh and Martinez (2000) note that mRET sacrifices some aspects of "loose training" to incorporate strategies that have been shown to facilitate speech production.

External scientific evidence

A number of researchers have evaluated the available evidence for treatment outcomes associated with RET and mRET. In general, positive outcomes have been associated with RET involving the use of picture description. Wambaugh, et al. (2012) determined that RET and mRET have shown positive outcomes on the production of content words for trained stimuli and generalization to untrained stimuli and contexts. Treatment effects have been maintained over time. The extent to which effects of RET or mRET generalize to untrained tasks and contexts may be relate to aphasia type, with non-fluent aphasia being associated with better generalization than fluent. Patients with a more severe anomia may also demonstrate poorer outcomes. RET has consistently resulted in improved production of content words in discourse. The authors conclude that RET has potential for clinical application since positive effects have been demonstrated with individuals with a variety aphasia types and severities.

Husak (2013) conducted a meta-analysis focusing on a "window of treatment" to examine RET from a "clinical perspective." Data was taken from 13 subjects with aphasia who participated in 12 RET studies that used picture stimuli. Husak calculated effect size for trained and untrained items. Positive treatment effects were evident after just 10 sessions, though the effects were larger with more treatment. Larger effect sizes were evident for patients with a more severe aphasia on trained and untrained items. Effect sizes for individual participants were medium or large for the majority of participants on both trained and untrained items.

Wisenburn et al. (2010) and Wisenburn (2011) conducted a meta-analysis of treatments for agrammatism that included two studies using mRET. The authors concluded that the results show a number of treatments, including mRET, have evidence for effectiveness in treating agrammatism. Wambaugh and Martinez (2000) demonstrated a medium effect size and Wambaugh et al. (2001) had a large effect size.

A search of the Clinical Aphasiology Conference proceedings resulted in 13 unique studies that referenced RET (http://aphasiology.pitt.edu/),
the majority of which were later published.
The American Speech-Language-Hearing Association (ASHA)
Practice Portal describes RET but provides no supporting evidence.
http://www.asha.org/PRPSpecificTopic.aspx?folderid=8589934663&section=Treatment
The ASHA Evidence Maps for aphasia do not specifically address RET.
http://www.ncepmaps.org/Aphasia-Treatment-Language-Oriented-Therapy.php
The Academy of Neurologic Communication Disorders and Sciences (ANCDS) developed evidence tables for studies on lexical retrieval, including RET. http://aphasiatx.arizona.edu/lexical

Clinical Expertise and Expert Opinion

A search for "response elaboration training" on the ASHA website produced 22 results, including 15 convention presentations suggesting a clinical interest in RET. Hinkley (2001) includes RET in review of conversational interventions. The single-subject studies reviewed for this guide included a total of 27 patients, all of whom demonstrated positive outcomes to varying degrees. The evidence suggests that picture description RET can increase the production of content words in trained and untrained contexts. The use of procedural prompts in lieu of pictures is promising, but the research is limited. The use of personal recounts is not currently supported by the research due to limited maintenance and generalization of treatment effects.

Patient and Caregiver Perspective

Wambaugh et al. (2012) report gains on measures of functional communication using the Communicative Effectiveness Index and the Communication Activities of Daily Living-2 for some patients. The majority of patients demonstrated minimal no change on self-perceptions of functional communication. The authors also note that two participants withdrew from treatment due to dislike of aspects of the treatment, particularly the 5 minutes of conversation required for the personal recount and the repetition of the task from day-to-day. Nessler and Wambaugh (2009) report modest gains on CETI for 2 patients with fluent aphasia.

Patients will vary in the extent to which they enjoy the flexible loose-training on which RET depends. Some patients may be more motivated to communicate if pictures depicting functional or interesting activities are used in place of low-context pictures.

References

Bennett, J., Wambaugh, J. L., & Nessler. (2005). Stimulus generalization effects of Response Elaboration Training. Paper presented at the Clinical Aphasiology Conference. Sanibel Island, FL.

http://aphasiology.pitt.edu/archive/00001543/01/95c05e71382f24e2304c0d831b00.pdf

Gaddie, A., Kearns, K. P., & Yedor, K. (1989). A qualitative analysis of Response Elaboration Training. Paper presented at the Clinical Aphasiology Conference. Lake Tahoe, CA.

http://aphasiology.pitt.edu/archive/00000113/01/19-17.pdf

Hinckley, J. J., Bourgeois, M. S., & Hickey, E. M. (2011). Treatments that work for both dementia and aphasia. Paper presented at the American Speech Language and Hearing Convention. San Diego, CA.

www.asha.org/Events/convention/handouts/2011/Hinckley-Bourgeois-Hickey/

Husak, R. S. (2013). Assessing the responsiveness to RET by individuals with chronic non-fluent aphasia: A clinical perspective. Paper presented at the Clinical Aphasiology Conference. Tucson, AZ.

http://aphasiology.pitt.edu/archive/00002440/01/Assessing_Responsiveness_to_RET_by_Individuals_with_Chronic_Non-fluent_Aphasia_A_Clinical_Perspective.pdf

Husak, R. S. and Marshall, R. C. (2012). Quantifying syntactic effects of Response Elaboration Training. Paper presented at the American Speech Language and Hearing Convention. San Diego, CA.

www.asha.org/Events/convention/handouts/2012/5122-Quantifying-Syntactic-Effects-of-Response-Elaboration-Training/

Kearns, K. P. (1985). Response Elaboration Training for patient initiated utterances. Paper presented at the Clinical Aphasiology Conference. Ashland, OR.

http://aphasiology.pitt.edu/archive/00000854/01/15-25.pdf

Kearns, K. P., & Scher, G. P. (1988). The generalization of Response Elaboration Training effects. Paper presented at the Clinical Aphasiology Conference. Cape Cod, MA.

http://aphasiology.pitt.edu/archive/00000076/01/18-17.pdf

Nessler, C., Wambaugh, J. L., & Wright, S. (2009). Effects of Response Elaboration Training on increased length and complexity of utterances with two participants with fluent aphasia. Paper presented at the Clinical Aphasiology Conference. Keystone, CO.

http://aphasiology.pitt.edu/archive/00002079/01/viewpaper.pdf

Nicholas, L. W., & Brookshire, R. H. (1993). A system for quantifying the informativeness and efficiency of the connected speech of adults with aphasia. *Journal of Speech and Hearing Research*, 36, 338–350. http://jslhr.pubs.asha.org/article.aspx?articleid=1779418

Rosenbek, J. C., Lemme, M. L., Ahern, M. B., Harris, E. H., & Wertz, R. (1973). A treatment for apraxia of speech in adults. *Journal of Speech and Hearing Disorders*, 38, 462-472. http://jshd.pubs.asha.org/article.aspx?articleid=1782878

Rosenbek, J. C., & Wertz, R. (1972). Treatment of apraxia of speech in adults. Paper presented at the Clinical Aphasiology Conference. Albuquerque, NM.

http://aphasiology.pitt.edu/archive/00000662/01/02-17.pdf

Wambaugh, J. L. (2000). Effects of Modified Response Elaboration Training with apraxic and aphasic speakers. *Aphasiology*, 14(5/6), 603-617.

Wambaugh, J. (2007). Acquired apraxia of speech: Current issues in management. Paper presented at the Texas Speech Language Hearing Association Meeting. Houston, TX.

http://www.txsha.org/_pdf/pdf/Wambaugh,%20Julie-Acquired%20Apraxia%20of%20Speech.pdf

Wambaugh, J. L., Martinez, A. L., & Alegre, M. N. (2001). Qualitative changes following application of Modified Response Elaboration Training with apraxic-aphasic speakers. *Aphasiology*, 15(10-11), 965-976.

Wambaugh, J. L., Nessler, C., & Wright, S. (2012). Response Elaboration Training: Application to procedural discourse and personal recounts. Paper presented at the Clinical Aphasiology Conference. Lake Tahoe, CA.

http://aphasiology.pitt.edu/archive/00002364/01/202-498-1-RV_%28Wambaugh_Nesser_Wright%29.pdf

Wambaugh, J. L., Nessler, C., & Wright, S. (2013). Modified Response Elaboration Training: Application to procedural discourse and personal recounts. *American Journal of Speech-Language Pathology*, 22(2), S409-S425.

http://ajslp.pubs.asha.org/Article.aspx?articleid=1795754

Wambaugh, J. L., Wright, S., & Nessler, C. (2012). Modified response elaboration training: A systematic extension with replications. *Aphasiology*, 26(12), 1407-1439.

Wisenburn, B. (2010). A meta-analysis of the therapy efficacy of agrammatism due to Aphasia. Paper presented at the American Speech Language and Hearing Convention. Philadelphia, PA.

www.asha.org/Events/convention/handouts/2010/1163-Wisenburn-Bruce/

Yedor, K., Conlon, C., & Kearns, K. P. (1991). Measurements predictive of generalization of Response Elaboration Training. Paper presented at the Clinical Aphasiology Conference. Destin, FL.

http://aphasiology.pitt.edu/archive/00001452/01/21-21.pdf

###

III - REDUCING APHASIC PERSEVERATION (RAP)

Reducing Aphasic Perseveration (RAP)

Purpose:

RAP is designed to reduce the occurrence of verbal perseveration on trained and untrained naming stimuli with generalization to conversational discourse. The goal is NOT to increase naming accuracy, though this may occur.

Intended Population:

RAP was designed for adults with acquired aphasia who demonstrate frequent perseveration. RAP has been used with patients who perseverate on 30% or more of items on a naming test. Patients may exhibit expressive and receptive language impairments but must have sufficient auditory comprehension and cognitive skills to understand the purpose of the treatment. RAP is not recommended for patients with severe global aphasia.

Anticipated Outcomes:

The treatment is associated with a reduction in the frequency of perseveration on trained and untrained naming tasks with generalization to discourse.

Administer a test of confrontation naming, such as the Boston Naming Test, which uses stimuli that will not be trained. Additionally, gather a short discourse sample to assess pre- and post-treatment occurrence of part- and whole-word perseverations.

Required Resources:

Pictures for naming task, stopwatch, pen, tracking sheets. SFA charts and ISI tracking sheets are available at http://www.recipeSLP.com.

Procedures

RAP treatment is fundamentally a picture naming activity that systematically manipulates the time between the presentation of each picture in a target set to gradually reduce the activation of the perseveration and seeks to strengthen the activation of the target using Semantic Feature Analysis (SFA). SFA treatment is a picture naming activity that uses a graphic organizer of semantic features to cue production of the target words. The clinician systematically facilitates identification of the semantic features of each target while facilitating the patient's ability to say the word (for additional information on SFA see *The Clinician's Guide to Semantic Feature Analysis for Aphasia*).

Candidacy for RAP treatment is determined based on patients' performance on a naming test. RAP appears to benefit patients who produce perseverative responses on 30% or more of items on a naming test.

Stimuli Selection

Since the goal of RAP is NOT naming accuracy, the same set of pictures can be used with each client. The words can be, but do not have to be, functional. Create three sets of five words and three sets of 10 words. The sets of five words can be used with more severe patients in order to repeat the treatment cycle as often as possible during a session. The larger sets can be used with less severe patients or as a patient shows improvement. The same set should be repeated until criterion for mastery is met.

When creating a treatment set, consider the semantic and phonological similarity between the target words: the greater the similarity, the greater the difficulty level. The first RAP treatment set should consist of words taken from a variety of semantic categories in order to reduce interference. If the patient improves but continues to exhibit perseverations, then training semantically related targets may provide a beneficial challenge.

A number of websites provide free access to picture stimuli that can be downloaded and printed to create treatment sets.

• The International Picture Naming Project offers 244 publically available object pictures.
http://crl.ucsd.edu/experiments/ipnp/method/getpics/getpics.html

• The Amsterdam Library of Object Images offers hundreds of color pictures for download.
http://aloi.science.uva.nl/

• Bonin et al., have made available a set of 299 black-and-white line drawings.
http://leadserv.u-bourgogne.fr/bases/pictures/

Before beginning treatment, design or select an SFA chart to guide the description of each target word. The features to be identified include: Group, Use, Action, Properties, Location, and Association. A number of versions of an SFA are available in the literature. SFA charts in English and Spanish are provided with the supplemental materials and are available for download at http://www.recipeSLP.com.

Define Perseveration

Before starting treatment, define perseveration for the participant and caregiver(s). Tell them that the patient gets stuck on a word and that the other words are weak and cannot come out. Use an analogy (verbal and graphic) of a light bulb that will not turn off (the perseveration) and a bulb that is too dim (the target) to explain the concept. Communicate that the purpose of the treatment is to turn off the perseveration and strengthen the target (e.g. make the light brighter) to make it easier for the patient to say what he/she really means.

The RAP Treatment Cycle

Treatment is a two-part cycle. Part 1 manipulates the interstimulus interval (ISI) between the presentations of pictures on a confrontation naming task. ISI refers to the time between presenting one picture and then the next picture. Part 2 involves conducting Semantic Feature Analysis (SFA; Boyle and Coelho, 1995) for any items that the patient did not name during Part 1 (regardless of perseveration).

The clinician repeats the two-part cycle as many times as possible in a session and from session to session, adjusting ISI as appropriate, until the criterion for mastery is met.

Part 1: ISI Manipulation

1. Present the first picture and ask the patient "What is this?"

2. Patient responds.

3. Once the patient indicates his/her response is complete (verbally or non-verbally), the ISI begins. If the patient perseverated in his attempt to name the picture, then add 2 seconds to the previous ISI. If the patient did not perseverate, then decrease the ISI by 2 seconds (regardless of accuracy).

4. Present the next picture.

5. Repeat steps 2 and 3 until all pictures in the set have been presented.

6. Move to SFA.

Part 2: Semantic Feature Analysis

1. Place the picture in the center of the SFA chart.

2. Ask the patient to name the picture-- "What is this?" (Do not name the picture).

3. Regardless of accuracy, guide the patient through the process of verbalizing the following features of the target: Group, Use, Action, Properties, Location, and Association.

4. Use a question, a sentence completion cue, or a choice to elicit the first feature, Group: "What category does it belong to?" "It is a type of _____." "Is it ___ or ___?" "Does it ____ or ___?"

5. Reinforce the feature by saying it and writing it on the chart.

6. Repeat for each feature.

7. If the chart is completed and the patient has not named the picture provide a phonological cue. If the patient still has not named the picture then say the name and ask the patient to repeat it.

8. Review the features of the target word.

9. Use the features to form a sentence. Tell the patient "A ____ is ____." (pointing to the features) "You say it. A ____ is ____."

10. The patient repeats the sentence.

11. Use the features to form a second sentence. Tell the patient "I ____ with a ____." (pointing to the features) "You say it. I ____ with a ____."

12. The patient repeats the sentence.

13. Repeat Steps 1-12 for each picture in the set that was not named in the ISI.

14. Return to the ISI activity. Begin with the ISI at which the previous cycle ended.

Homework

Train the caregiver on the treatment procedure when possible. Provide the training words and corresponding pictures as well as the ISI reached at the end of each treatment session. Instruct the caregiver and patient to complete the treatment activity at least once each day. Encourage them to talk about and describe the objects pictured.

Important Tips for ISI Manipulation and SFA:

• For the very first session, begin with an ISI of 20 second or at the ISI best for the patient.

• The ISI required to consistently eliminate perseverations will vary widely. In the initial sessions, the ISI may repeatedly increase until the right ISI for the patient is reached.

• Use a timer or stopwatch to monitor the ISI but be aware that the timing of the ISI will not be exact for a number of reasons. Generally, the range of ISI should steadily shift to shorter intervals.

• Each cycle is considered a fresh start in counting perseveration. Do not count a word as a perseveration until it is repeated in the same cycle. The only exception is the production of habitual perseverations (e.g. words that the patient perseverates on across a variety of contexts).

• "No response" is considered an acceptable response since the patient did not perseverate.

• Change the order of the items presentation for each cycle.

• If the patient does not say the whole- or part-word perseveration but visible groping suggests that the patient is attempting to suppress the perseveration do not count this response as a perseveration.

Criterion for Mastery

A set is mastered when the patient produces no perseverations on 9/10 or 4/5 target words with an ISI <2 seconds.

After Set 1 is mastered, probe Set 2. If the patient's perseveration rate is less than or equal to 10% on the Set 2 probe, then he/she may be ready to continue with a different treatment. Re-administer pre-testing naming and discourse tasks to measure outcomes and generalization.

Tracking performance

ISI should be tracked on an item by item basis for each cycle. Use this information to know the ISI for the first item in the next cycle and to determine if criterion for mastery has been met. You also may choose to track accuracy to measure improvement in naming.

RAP in Action

Below is an example of a typical client-clinician exchange during the ISI portion of the RAP Cycle. Assume the last RAP cycle ended with an ISI of 32 seconds and that the patient habitually perseverates on the word "hat." Note that the ISI is increased when the patient says "hat" because it is a habitual perseveration. The ISI is not increased the first time the patient says "duck" because he/she did not say the word when the picture of the duck was presented. The ISI is increased the second time the patient says "duck."

Clinician: What is this? [shows the patient the first picture, house]

Patient: Uhh, hat, no. [shakes head]

Clinician: OK, let's move on. Just clear your mind. [Remove picture from field of vision and wait quietly for 34 seconds.]

Clinician: What is this? [shows the patient the second picture, duck]

Patient: [visible groping, shakes head].

Clinician: Great. Just clear your mind. [Remove picture from field of vision. Wait quietly for 32 seconds.]

Clinician: What is this? [shows the patient the third picture, apple]

Patient: Uhmm, duck.

Clinician: OK, let's move on. Just clear your mind. [Remove picture from field of vision. Wait quietly for 30 seconds.]

Clinician: What is this? [shows the patient the third picture, blouse].

Patient: Uhmm, duck.

Clinician: OK. Just clear your mind. [Remove picture from field of vision. Wait quietly for 32 seconds.]

Clinician: What is this? [shows the patient the fourth picture]

Below is an example of a typical client-clinician exchange during the SFA portion of the RAP cycle. Note that the action category is skipped because in the case of the target word "television" action and use are closely tied. Patients who perseverate often have difficulty producing the descriptors so quite a bit of support is provided.

The clinician shows the patient a picture of a television.

Clinician: What is this?

Patient: Uhh, yeah. [points to eyes]

Clinician: It's something you watch?

Patient: Yeah, yeah.

Clinician: It's something you watch. [writes "watch" in USE category]

Clinician: What group does it belong to?

Patient: Uhmmm. [shrugs shoulders and shakes head]

Clinician: Is it a kind of clothing or electronics?

Patient: Yeah, yeah. El— say again.

Clinician: Electronics. Right, it's a type of electronics. [writes "electronics" in GROUP category]

Clinician: You said you like to watch it. Is there anything else you use it for?

Patient: Uhh, no, hat…no.

Clinician: What is it like?

Patient: Well.. it's like a.. ..[makes shape of a rectangular with hands]

Clinician: It's shaped like a rectangle. Excellent. [writes "rectangle" in PROPERTIES box]

Clinician: Where do you find it?

Patient: Uhmm, yes, and no, and yes. [pointing as if to different rooms]

Clinician: You find it in some rooms but not others?

Patient: Yes, yes.

Clinician: Do you find it in the living room or the bathroom?

Patient: Li- li- live room.

Clinician: Excellent. You find it in the living room. [writes "living room" in the LOCATION box]

Clinician: It's like a _____.

Patient: Hummm [shakes head].

Clinician: Is it like a radio or a kettle?

Patient: Rayo.

Clinician: Great. It's like a radio. [writes "radio" in ASSOCIATION box]

Clinician: [Pointing to each box in turn] So you said it's a type of electronics that you watch. It is rectangular. You can find it in the living room and it's like a radio.

Clinician: [Pointing to picture] What is this?

Patient: Uhh, uhhh. [shakes head]

Clinician: It's a te-.

Patient: Te- te- telelision.

Clinician: Close. Television. You say it.

Patient: Television.

Clinician: Great. Television. A television is a type of electronics you use to watch shows that is rectangular. You have one in your living room and it's like a radio. What is this? [pointing to picture]

Patient: Umm tel- tel-....

Clinician: Television.

Patient: Television.

Clinician: Let's use it in a sentence. "A television is in the living room. You say it. A television is in the living room." [pointing to the feature on the chart]

Patient: Television living room.

Clinician: A television is in the living room. Let's try another one. I watch a television. You say it. I watch television. [pointing to the feature on the chart]

Patient: I, uhh, uhh.

Clinician: Listen, again. I watch television.

Patient: I watch television.

Clinician: Excellent. Are you ready for the next one?

Cues, Supports, and Modifications

RAP can be modified in a number of ways to make the task easier or harder based on the patient's level of functioning. The following supports can be provided as needed.

During ISI Manipulation:

• Wait quietly and ask the patient to relax and clear his/her mind.

• DO NOT do any of the following: talk about perseveration, repeat the perseveration, instruct the patient not to perseverate, or comment on visible oral groping.

• DO NOT tell the patient the target response.

• Discourage rehearsal of the target. Remove the picture of the target to avoid continued efforts by the patient to say the name of the object.

During Semantic Feature Analysis:

• Provide appropriate cues and support for SFA to assist the patient in working through the process more quickly.

• Read the question and point to the appropriate section of the graphic organizer.

• Write the feature in the appropriate section of the graphic organizer.

• Provide choices to help the patient identify the features (e.g. "Is it a food or furniture?").

• Tell the patient the feature.

• Point to features written on the graphic organizer to help the patient complete the cloze sentences.

• Model the cloze sentence and ask the patient to repeat it.

Using RAP with Spanish speakers:

• Use the RAP procedures as described (see Spanish SFA chart below).

• Select stimuli that are represented by a single word in Spanish.

• Select stimuli that should be familiar to Spanish speakers.

• Use the following phonological cuing hierarchy when needed: article (el/la), syllabic cue (rather than phonemic cue), provide the word.

• The Spanish SFA chart and five stimuli lists are provided with the supplemental materials and available for download at http://www.recipeslp.com. Each list includes 10 words balanced for frequency and number of syllables. Set 1 includes el cocodrilo, el pato, el labio, la iglesia, el abrigo, el pastel, la sandilla, la mariposa, el reloj, la olla. Set 2 includes la ardilla, el búho, el cabello, la cerca, el vestido, la naranja, el escritorio, la abeja, el salero, la uva.

A Summary of the Theory and Evidence

The EBP Triangle

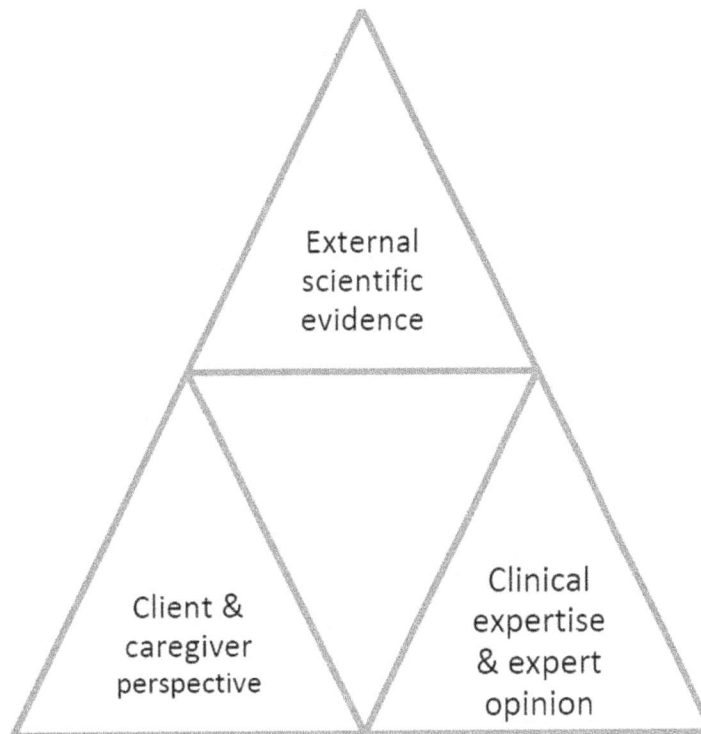

Theory

RAP was developed from a theoretical understanding of perseveration and lexical access. According to an activation model of lexical access, perseverations result from the over and persistent activation of a recently spoken word or habitual response. Two components are needed to produce a perseveration: persistent activation of a previous response and weak activation (phonological and/or semantic) of the target response (Cohen & Dehaene, 1998; Martin & Dell, 2007). The interaction of these two processes results in the production of the perseveration rather than the target. RAP is designed to increase activation of the target while systematically decreasing the time required to deactivate the perseverative response.

External Scientific Evidence

The evidence to guide treatment for perseveration is extremely limited (Stark, 2011). The author completed two case studies measuring the outcomes obtained from RAP (Muñoz, 2011; Muñoz, in review). Both patients decreased perseveration to zero or near zero on trained and untrained naming tasks. One patient reached criterion on the first training set in seven sessions. A decrease in part-word and whole-word repletion was evident in measures of narrative discourse. Additionally, the decline in perseverations was maintained over time.

Semantic Feature Analysis, as an independent treatment, has been studied by a number of researchers with positive outcomes. See RecipeSLP's *The SLP's Guide to Semantic Feature Analysis* for more information.

Clinical Expertise and Expert Opinion

Expert opinion differs on the issue of whether or not perseverations should be targeted directly or indirectly. Basso (2004) argues that perseverations, like other paraphasias, are a symptom of the underlying disruption in lexical retrieval. Treating the impairment in the phonological or semantic system directly will indirectly reduce the occurrence of perseveration. While this point is valid, clinical experience suggests that for some patients with significant perseverations, helping them eliminate the perseverations first frees up the lexical system to produce other types of responses, though the responses may still be incorrect. Semantic or phonological paraphasias provide the listener with more clues about the intended lexical target than do perseverations.

Patient and Caregiver Perspective

The patients reported in the case studies (Muñoz, 2011; Muñoz in review) both understood the concept of perseveration and quickly endeavored to suppress the perseveration. Though the time required to complete the treatment varied, both patients demonstrated sustained and generalized reduction in perseveration. The caregivers of both patients reported an increase in how much the patient was able to communicate and the quality of their communicative relationship.

References

Basso, A. (2004). Perseveration or the tower of Babel. *Seminars in Speech and Language, 25* (4), 375-389.

Boyle, M., & Coelho, C. A. (1995). Application of semantic feature analysis as a treatment for aphasic dysnomia. *American Journal of Speech-Language Pathology, 4*, 94-98. http://ajslp.pubs.asha.org/article.aspx?articleid=1774521

Cohen, L., & Dehaene, S. (1998). Competition between past and present: Assessment and interpretation of verbal perseverations. *Brain, 121*, 1641-1659.

Dell, G. S., Burger, L. K., & Svec, W. R. (1997). Language production and serial order: A functional analysis and a model. *Psychological Review, 104*(1), 123-147.

Muñoz, M. L. (2011). Reducing aphasic perseverations: A case study. *Perspectives on Neurophysiology and Neurogenic Speech and Language Disorders, 21*(4), 176-183. http://sig2perspectives.pubs.asha.org/article.aspx?articleid=1768798

Muñoz, M.L. (in review). A treatment to reduce aphasic perseveration. Submitted to *Aphasiology*.

Stark, J. (2011). Treatment of verbal perseveration in persons with aphasia. *Perspectives on Neurophysiology and Neurogenic Speech and Language Disorders, 21*(4), 152-166. http://sig2perspectives.pubs.asha.org/article.aspx?articleid=1768796

###

46

Supplimental Materials

What group does it belong to?	How do you use it?	What does it do?

← Target Item

What is it like?	Where do you find it?	What does it remind you of?

¿En qué grupo se encuentra?	¿Para qué se usa?	¿Qué hace?

Objeto

¿Come es?	¿Dónde se encuentra?	¿De qué le recuerda?

What group does it belong to?	How do you use it?	What does it do?

← Target Item

What is it like?	Where do you find it?	What does it remind you of?

1. A _____ is _____.
2. I _____ with a _____.

¿En qué grupo se encuentra?	¿Para qué se usa?	¿Qué hace?

Objeto ←

¿Come es?	¿Dónde se encuentra?	¿De qué le recuerda?

1. Un _____ es _____ .

2. Yo _____ con el _____ .

RET Tracking Sheet

Target	Patient's initial response to each picture	# content words in initial response	# content words in final elaborated response
	Total		
	Average		

Spanish word lists for Reducing Aphasic Perseveration

Set 1	Syllables		Set 4	Syllables
El Cocodrilo	4		El león	2
El pato	2		El gallo	2
El labio	2		La oreja	3
La iglesia	4		La puerta	2
El abrigo	3		El calcetín	3
El pastel	2		La alcachofa	4
La sandilla	3		La fresa	2
La mariposa	4		La silla	2
El reloj	2		El saltamontes	4
La olla	2		La estufa	3
	2.8			2.7

Set 2			Set 5	
La ardilla	3		El vendado	3
El búho	2		El avestruz	3
El cabello	3		La mano	2
La cerca	2		La cerradura	4
El vestido	3		La falda	2
La naranja	3		La calabaza	4
El escritorio	5		La pina	2
La abeja	3		El tocador	3
El salero	3		La mosca	2
La uva	2		El hervidor	3
	2.9			2.8

Set 3	
La cabra	2
La águila	3
La pierna	2
La ventana	3
El gorro	2
El elote	3
El cacahuate	4
El cenicero	4
La oruga	3
La canasta	3

RAP Tracking Sheet

	Target	Correct/ Incorrect	Time (Sec.)	Picture Naming Response	P

Missed Items	Responsiveness to Semantic Feature Analysis

About Recipe SLP

Recipe SLP, EBP how-to for SLPs, is the speech-language pathologist's source for affordable guides to the science and practice behind clinical procedures for managing communication impairments across the lifespan. We examine the literature in order to report the purpose, target population, and foundational steps for each procedure. Additionally, we explain variations and modifications that can expand the usefulness of the procedure. Based on our own clinical experience, we provide tips, suggestions, and sample exchanges to help clinicians feel confident when implementing the treatment procedures. Each guide includes a brief up-to-date summary of the evidence supporting each treatment and a bibliography with active links to online research articles, conference presentations, and relevant websites.

Recipe SLP is committed to helping speech-language pathologists transfer knowledge between science and practice. Our books summarize the methods and evidence for procedures used by speech-language pathologists to address communication challenges resulting from impairments in speech, language, and cognition across the lifespan. Recipe SLP values culturally relevant practice in speech-language pathology and considers the applicability of the clinical procedures for culturally and linguistically diverse populations.

We would love to hear from you!

Visit our website http://www.recipeslp.com
Like us on Facebook https://www.facebook.com/recipeSLP
Follow us on Twitter https://twitter.com/RecipeSLP
Read our blog http://recipeslp.wordpress.com/

More books by Recipe SLP

The Aphasia Series
The Clinician's Guide to Semantic Feature Analysis
The Clinician's Guide to Reducing Aphasic Perseveration
The Aphasia Series Vol. 1: SFA, RET, RAP

About the Author

Nearly 25 years of experience as a speech-language pathologist has given Maria L. Muñoz, Ph.D., CCC-SLP insight into the profession from the perspective of a student, a clinician, a researcher, a clinical supervisor, and an instructor. Her commitment to engage in and teach evidence-based practice led her to two questions: How do clinicians find the time and resources needed for EBP? Where do clinicians go to learn how to implement specific treatments? Not finding good answers to either question, she came up with one…Recipe SLP, the SLP's source for affordable guides to the science and practice behind clinical procedures for managing communication impairments across the lifespan.

Dr. Muñoz is currently an associate professor in Fort Worth, TX. She earned her Ph.D. from the University of Texas at Austin as a participant in the Multicultural Leadership Training Program, after which she completed a post-doctoral fellowship at the University of Arizona. Dr. Muñoz has clinical experience working with adults and children with impairments in speech, language, and cognition. She teaches and provides clinical supervision in the area of acquired neurologically-based disorders of language and cognition in adults, particularly individuals who are Spanish speaking or bilingual. Additionally, she teaches courses related to the management of communication disorders in culturally and linguistically diverse individuals across the life span and a course in counseling individuals with communication impairments and their families. She conducts research on aphasia in bilinguals and Spanish speakers, as well as pedagogy in communication sciences and disorders. Her work has been published in a number of peer-reviewed journals including *Aphasiology*, *American Journal of Speech-Language Pathology*, and *Brain and Language*.